Treating Obesity

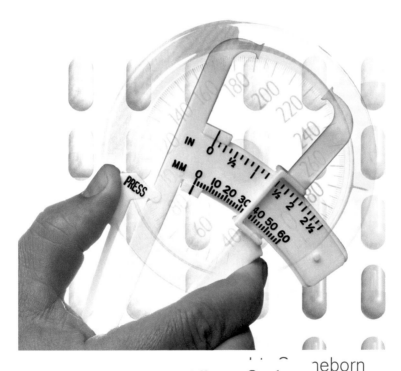

Liz Sonneborn

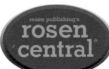

rosen publishing's
rosen central®

New York

Published in 2009 by The Rosen Publishing Group, Inc.
29 East 21st Street, New York, NY 10010

First Edition

Library of Congress Cataloging-in-Publication Data

Sonneborn, Liz.
Treating obesity / Liz Sonneborn.
    p. cm.—(Understanding obesity)
Includes bibliographical references and index.
ISBN-13: 978-1-4042-1771-3 (library binding)
1. Obesity—Treatment. I. Title.
RC628.S682 2009
616.3'9806—dc22

                                        20070518041

Manufactured in the United States of America

Contents

Introduction

Every year it's the same. On December 31, millions of Americans make resolutions to change something in their lives. And, for many of them, there is one resolution that makes the list year after year—the promise finally to do something about their excess weight.

For some, that might mean trying to take off 5 or 10 pounds (2.3 or 4.5 kilograms). To reach their goal, they might cut back on sweets and exercise a little more. In a few months' time and with a little effort, their clothes will be fitting looser.

But for many others, losing weight is not that simple. It is especially hard for those who are obese. Generally, people are considered obese if their bodies have an excessive amount of body fat—the tissue that contains stores of energy.

For slightly overweight people, the primary motivation for losing weight is their appearance. In American culture, lean, toned bodies are seen as attractive. Getting rid of a few extra pounds is likely to earn compliments from others and to increase a person's own self-assurance and confidence. Obese people have an additional reason for slimming down. Just as our society praises the thin, it punishes the obese. Almost from birth, Americans are schooled in stereotypes about the severely overweight. They are branded as ugly, lazy, and utterly lacking in self-control. And they suffer enormously from these preconceptions. Obese children are tortured by bullies. Obese teenagers are scorned by their peers. Obese adults are faced with discrimination on a daily basis,

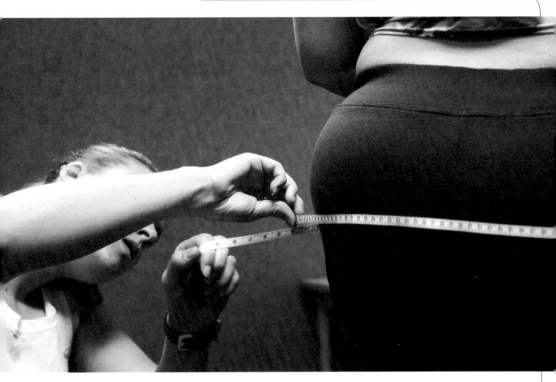

A teenager at the Carnegie International Camp in Bradford, England, has her hip measurement taken as part of a weekly assessment. For many dieters, a tape measure and a scale are useful tools for measuring their weight-loss progress.

affecting every aspect of their lives. The stigma of obesity can take an enormous toll, often leading to depression and despair.

As awful as the prejudices against obese people are, many face something far worse—living with the chronic and even life-threatening health problems that have been linked to obesity. According to the Centers for Disease Control and Prevention (CDC), the federal agency charged with protecting public health, obese people are at risk for high blood pressure, osteoarthritis, type 2 diabetes, heart disease, stroke, gallbladder disease, sleep apnea, and some cancers. This news is certainly alarming for obese individuals. But it also has dire implications for American society. Since the 1980s, the United States has seen a sharp increase in obesity rates. With more of the population prone to developing obesity-related health problems, the emotional, societal, and financial costs of caring for the sick is a growing burden.

Treating obesity, therefore, is important to people suffering from the stress and dangers of severe weight problems. But it also affects every American. As obesity rates are rising in many parts of the world, eventually it will likely impact nearly everyone on the planet.

Some people are dismissive about the plight of the obese. They laugh off the struggle to lose weight, counseling the obese to simply eat less and exercise more. In reality, though, treating obesity is not so easy. Even with hoards of scientific researchers and a multibillion-dollar diet industry searching for how to end obesity, it remains a complex, maddening problem—one that has ramifications for all of us.

Chapter 1

Calories In, Calories Out

There are several methods medical professionals can use to make precise measurements of body fat. For instance, they might X-ray the entire body (dual-energy X-ray absorptiometry) or weigh a person underwater (hydrostatic weighing). Both methods are fairly time-consuming and expensive. A simpler, but still reliable measure of body fat is body mass index, or BMI. A person's BMI is a number calculated by multiplying the person's weight in pounds by 703 (a correction factor), then dividing that number by the person's height in inches squared. For a quick way of determining a BMI, consult the Web site of the U.S. government's Centers for Disease Control and Prevention (CDC). It offers a BMI calculator for adults and one for children and adolescents (http://www.cdc.gov/nccdphp/dnpa/bmi/index.htm).

MEASURING OBESITY

Based on their BMI, adults can be classified as underweight, normal, overweight, or obese. The chart below shows these classifications as defined by the CDC.

BMI	Weight Status
Below 18.5	Underweight
18.5 to 24.9	Normal
25.0 to 29.9	Overweight
30.0 or more	Obese

Although this system is fairly accurate, in some cases it can place a person in the wrong category. A BMI often underestimates the amount of body fat in an elderly person, while it overestimates it in a very muscular athlete. For instance, according to a 2005 survey conducted by the Associated Press, nearly half of the players in the National Basketball Association (NBA) would be considered overweight based on their BMIs. The BMI of famed basketball star Shaquille O'Neal was so high that it identified him as being obese.

Even in those of normal weight, body fat can still pose a health problem. Health researchers have found that people with too much fat in their midsections are at risk for heart disease, diabetes, and high blood pressure. As a result, they urge people concerned about their weight to measure the circumference of their waist. According to the National Heart, Lung, and Blood Institute (NHLBI), a waist measuring more than 40 inches (102 centimeters) on a man or more than 35 inches (89 cm) on a woman puts that person at higher risk of having serious health problems.

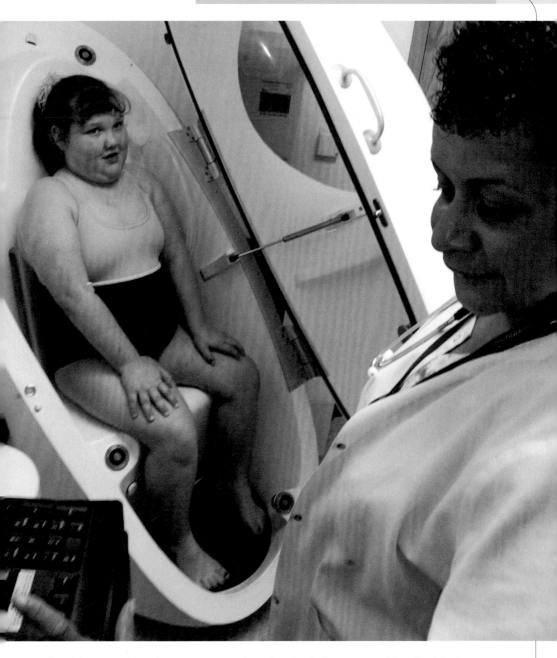

An eight-year-old patient prepares to have her body fat measured in a Bod Pod. Body fat can be estimated from a person's height and weight. But special medical devices such as the Bod Pod, which uses air displacement technology, can safely and quickly provide a more accurate measure.

SETTING GOALS

When, based on their BMI and waist circumference, people discover they need to lose weight, what should they do next? In 1998, a panel of experts at the NHLBI exhaustively examined this question. They put their findings in a brief report titled *The Practical Guide: Identification, Evaluation, and Treatment of Overweight and Obesity in Adults*. Ever since, doctors have used this report to set guidelines for their patients' weight loss.

The Practical Guide advises obese people to set an initial goal of losing 10 percent of their body weight over a period of six months. This rule is not always embraced by people hoping to lose more weight far quicker. But according to NHLBI's experts, a slow, steady weight loss is easier to maintain than a rapid drop. They recommend losing no more than 1 to 2 pounds (0.5 to 1 kg) per week.

With that goal in mind, *The Practical Guide* suggests people try to lose weight by limiting the amount of food energy they take in—in other words, to go on a low-calorie diet (LCD). (A calorie is a unit of measure equal to the amount of energy it takes to increase the temperature of 1 kilogram of water by 1 degree Celsius.) For dieters, it is important to know that 3,500 calories is equal to one pound (0.5 kg). Therefore, to lose one pound per week, a person's calorie intake has to be reduced by 500 calories per day (7 days x 500 calories = 3,500 calories).

The total number of calories a person should consume to reach that goal varies from person to person. But *The Practical Guide* offers general guidelines that will work for most people. It recommends that women on an LCD should eat between 1,000 and 1,200 calories daily, while men should consume between 1,200 and 1,600 calories per day.

Sometimes, doctors recommend a VLCD (very low-calorie diet) for obese people. These diets provide only 800 calories or less per day. No one should go on a VLCD casually because such severe restriction of calories can cause health problems. As a result, a person on a VLCD has to be carefully monitored by a doctor experienced in their use. A VLCD can help patients lose weight quickly, but they tend to quickly gain back every pound they lost if they go off the diet.

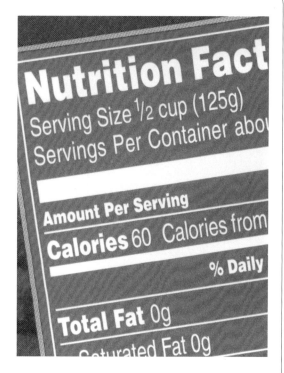

Food labels listing the number of calories per serving are a great help to people on low-calorie diets.

PLANNING A WEIGHT-LOSS STRATEGY

Doctors are not the only experts who can monitor a dieter's progress. Nutritionists and dietitians can also offer expertise to better ensure success. Many hospitals house weight-loss clinics that offer obese patients access to experts in a variety of fields.

For financial reasons, most people looking to lose weight have to educate themselves about low-calorie dieting. That is not an easy job. Dieters have to figure out the calorie content of favorite foods. They also have to learn to read food labels, to

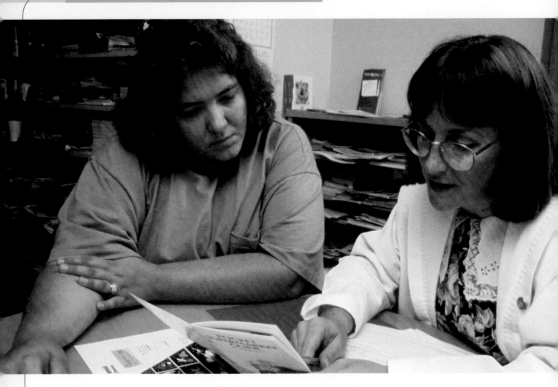

People wanting to lose weight can better their chances for success by consulting a dietician. Formally trained in food and nutrition science, dieticians can give advice about a dieter's ideal daily calorie intake and offer suggestions for choosing healthy and filling foods.

cook using lower-calorie ingredients, and to reduce the size of their portions at every meal.

For help, many dieters rely on diet books. While some are based on medically sound information, others are not. Some recommend fad diets that promise great results by making strange food choices. One famous fad diet advocates eating grapefruit and grapefruit juice at every meal. First developed in the 1930s in Hollywood, the grapefruit diet reemerges every few years, briefly attracting new enthusiasts until it again becomes clear that few dieters can stand eating that much grapefruit for very long.

In recent years, dieters have been able to purchase a wide variety of special diet foods. For example, at any grocery store, they can find meal replacement bars. One manufacturer of these bars suggests dieters eat one for breakfast, one for lunch, and then end the day with a "reasonable" dinner of their own choosing. Weight-loss experts generally frown on this type of meal replacement program. The bars might provide an adequate number of calories, but they do not stave off hunger well. By dinnertime, dieters are likely to be so ravenous that they cannot help themselves from eating an unreasonable amount of food.

Experts are more comfortable with the use of low-calorie frozen meals. They offer portion-controlled meals, usually of between 300 and 400 calories. For dieters new to calorie counting, these meals keep them from accidentally eating more than their low-calorie diet allows. Portion-controlled meals form the corner-stone of some commercial weight-loss programs, such as Jenny Craig and NutriSystem. These programs also offer some nutritional education, guidelines for exercise, and emotional support. They are, however, fairly expensive. Weight-loss researchers also complain that the reliance on preprepared meals often does not adequately prepare dieters for making wise food choices after they have reached their weight-loss goal.

LOW FAT VS. LOW CARBOHYDRATE

Technically, a calorie is a calorie. Suppose one person eats a healthy diet of 1,200 calories each day, while another eats nothing but 1,200 calories' worth of marshmallow fluff. Clearly, the marshmallow fluff eater will suffer a few stomachaches and probably some more dire health problems. But, if these two people

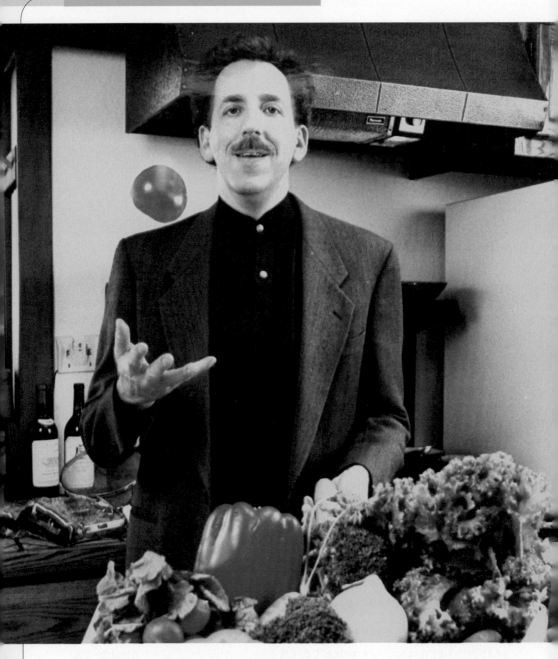

Dean Ornish is a well-known advocate for eating a diet that is very low in fat. Ornish not only recommends a low-fat diet for weight loss, but he also claims it can help prevent heart disease. To further study the effects of diet and lifestyle on disease, Ornish founded the Preventative Medicine Research Institute in 1986.

are starting from the same weight, they will lose the same number of pounds at the same rate. However, several of the most popular diets advocate the importance of food choice in losing weight and keeping it off for the long term. One type calls for limiting fats in the diet, while another insists on limiting carbohydrates.

Perhaps the most famous low-fat advocate is Dean Ornish, a professor of medicine at the University of California–San Francisco. He recommends eating a diet very low in fats, such as butter and oils. Most of the calories in his plan come from fruits, vegetables, whole grains, and a limited amount of low-fat proteins, such as fish and chicken. The title of his best-selling book *Eat More, Weigh Less* explains the biggest selling point of his low-fat diet. Dieters on the Ornish plan can eat relatively large quantities of filling low-fat foods, while still consuming fewer calories. As an added benefit, Ornish claims his plan is so heart-healthy that it can even reverse heart disease.

On the other side of the spectrum are low-carbohydrate diets. The most famous was developed by Robert Atkins in the 1960s. In 1972, he first published the details of his diet plan in the best-selling *Dr. Atkins' Diet Revolution*. Atkins claimed that carbohydrates were making people fat. These foods caused blood glucose (blood sugar) first to soar and then to crash. With the crash came intense hunger, making people overeat.

Based on this theory, Atkins's diet prohibits or limits most carbohydrates, including potatoes, pasta, white rice, white bread, carrots, corn, and watermelon. Instead, Atkins allows dieters to eat large amounts of fat and protein, including butter, steak, and bacon. In 2003 and 2004, the Atkins plan enjoyed a renewed burst of popularity. At the height of the Atkins craze, National

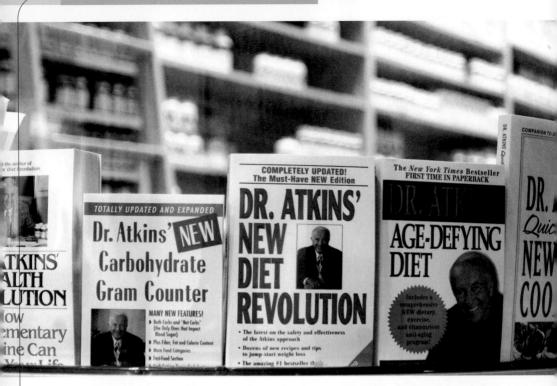

In recent years, many Americans have tried the controversial Atkins diet. First introduced in the 1970s, the Atkins plan calls for severely cutting back on carbohydrates, such as potatoes, white rice, and pasta, but allows dieters to eat large amounts of fat and protein.

Public Radio reported that an estimated one out of every eleven North Americans was on the diet. Enthusiasm for the Atkins diet has since faded, much to the relief of many health experts. They claimed the fatty diet would surely increase cholesterol levels, leading to a spike in heart disease.

In March 2007, the results of a Stanford University study of four diets, including Ornish's and Atkins's, was published in the *Journal of the American Medical Association*. Contrary to popular opinion in the medical community, the Atkins diet did not cause an increase in cholesterol levels. In addition, it offered dieters the largest weight loss of all four diets examined. But even so, the

Myths and Facts

Myth: All fat-free foods are low in calories.
Fact: Some fat-free foods are fairly low in calories, but many are not. Sometimes, because of added sugar, a fat-free product actually has more calories than the full-fat version.

Myth: Skipping meals is a good way to lose weight.
Fact: Skipping meals, especially breakfast, can set up dieters for disaster. If dieters allow themselves to get too hungry, chances are they will overeat at their next meal.

Myth: Eating after seven o'clock at night makes people gain weight.
Fact: It does not matter when people eat. Excess calories will be stored as fat regardless of what time of day they are consumed.

weight loss achieved on the Atkins diet was hardly impressive. After a year on the plan, Atkins dieters lost an average of only 10 pounds (4.5 kg). Those on the other diets studied lost an even more dismal 3 to 6 pounds (1.4 to 2.7 kg).

In this way, the study pointed out the sad truth known to many dieters. The number of people on diets who succeed at losing weight and keeping it off is low. In fact, the CDC reports that 98 percent of people who try to lose weight fail. For most people, dieting is not enough to make a lasting change. But, as the next chapter will show, there are some things those truly committed to lifetime weight loss can do to beat the odds.

Chapter 2

Beyond Dieting

In 1993, medical researchers James Hill and Rena Wing founded the National Weight Control Registry. They began collecting data on people who had lost 30 pounds (13.6 kg) and kept them off more than a year. They discovered that there was no one diet that seemed to work better than the rest. The people in the registry had lost weight using all sorts of diet strategies, but they did have one thing in common: virtually all of them had incorporated regular physical activity into their lives.

MAKING AN EXERCISE REGIME

The finding was hardly surprising. Experts generally recommend that people on low-calorie diets also begin an exercise regimen. According to the NHLBI, "All adults should set a long-term goal to accumulate at least thirty minutes or more of

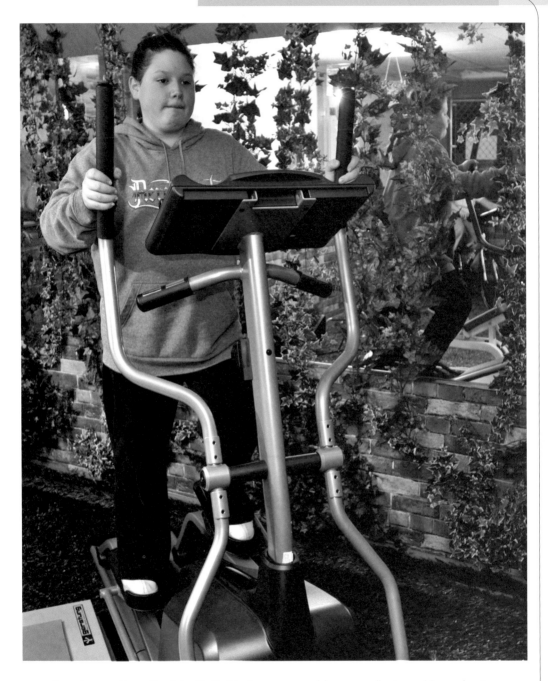

Exercise machines, like this elliptical trainer, can provide an excellent aerobic workout, whether at a gym or at home. A well-rounded exercise program should also include strength training to build muscle and stretching to promote flexibility.

Exercise Basics

A good exercise program includes three types of physical activity—aerobic exercise, strength training, and stretching. Aerobic exercise raises the breathing rate and makes the heart pump faster. It also burns calories. Examples include walking, running, swimming, and roller-skating. Strength training, which usually involves lifting weights, builds stronger muscles. It also helps people to lose weight. The more muscular a person is, the more calories he or she burns even at rest. Stretching or activities such as yoga or Pilates keep joints flexible. Flexibility reduces a person's chance of injury while enjoying other physical activities.

moderate-intensity physical activity on most, and preferably all, days of the week."

For the obese, this amount of physical activity can seem daunting. At least at first, obese people may find even moderate exercise exhausting, and they may be prone to injury. With this in mind, experts recommend that obese people start slowly when beginning an exercise program, working up to thirty minutes each day over time. They often suggest obese patients initially take up aerobic walking because it is safe and simple to do.

Some people find it difficult to put aside half an hour each day just for exercise. But according to the NHLBI, studies show that daily exercise does not have to be performed in one thirty-minute block. Exercising in ten-minute spurts three times per day will provide the same health benefits.

When beginning an exercise program, many people assume they need to join a gym to see results. Over the long haul, working out at home is probably the best option for most people. Having a treadmill, dumbbells, or other equipment in sight acts as a cue, reminding people they need to exercise. Dieters who cannot find the time for formal workout sessions should instead try to increase the physical activity in their everyday lives. For instance, weight-loss professionals often suggest people take stairs instead of an elevator, or park a distance away from their destination to force themselves to walk more.

While exercise is generally recommended as part of any obesity treatment, it is not the whole answer. Very few people can lose large amounts of weight with exercise alone. The reason why is simple: it takes a great deal of exercise to burn a substantial number of calories. For instance, walking 1 mile (1.6 kilometers) at a moderate pace (fifteen to twenty minutes) burns about 100 calories. Therefore, to lose just 1 pound (0.5 kg) by walking alone, an average person would need to walk 35 miles (56 km).

BEHAVIORAL MODIFICATION

Another common component in treating obesity is behavioral therapy. Weight-loss experts have identified several tried-and-true techniques for changing dieters' behavior in ways that will help them eat less. For instance, doctors will often use a technique called shaping. This involves working with an obese patient to select a series of weight-loss goals. The doctor then writes down

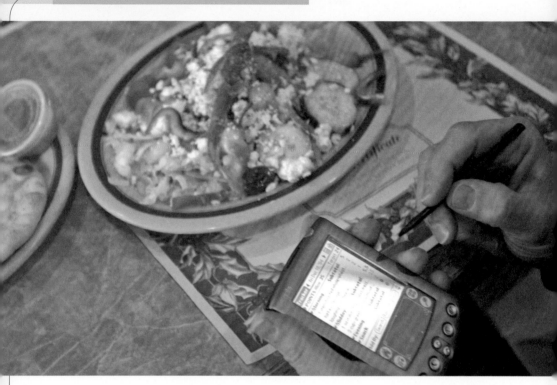

A dieter records what he has eaten for lunch on a personal digital assistant (PDA). Whether kept on an electronic device or in a notebook, a food diary can help prevent people on weight-loss programs from accidentally overeating.

these goals and gives them to the patient. This "prescription" can help keep patients on track by reminding them of their weight-loss plan.

Another behavior-changing technique is identifying stimuli—this is something a person sees or does that triggers eating. A common example is watching television. People who realize that they always eat more at meals if the television is on can vow to turn it off during dinner.

Studies have found that even small changes in behavior can make a difference. For some people, just keeping a daily diary of the food they eat can help them consume less. For others, using a smaller plate can trick them into thinking their portion size is larger than it is. One common behavior modification is consciously trying to eat at a slower pace or using the nondominant hand to eat (that is, using your left hand to eat if you are usually right-handed). It takes about twenty minutes for the stomach to tell the brain it is full. By eating more slowly, people are less likely to keep eating past the point of fullness.

When trying to lose weight, many people have greater success if they have the support of other dieters. They may seek support of friends who are also struggling with their weight, or they can chat with other dieters on Internet message boards. Some commercial weight-loss plans, such as Weight Watchers, use support groups to help motivate their customers. Two national not-for-profit organizations—Overeaters Anonymous and Take Off Pounds Sensibly (TOPS)—also offer group support meetings at little or no cost.

DRUG THERAPY

For some people trying to lose weight, particularly those classified as obese, dieting, even when combined with exercise and behavior modification, is not enough. They may find it impossible to get close to their weight-loss goals. For these people, doctors sometimes recommend medical treatments developed for combating obesity.

If a patient with a BMI above 30 has failed to lose weight though diet and exercise over a six-month period, a doctor may prescribe a weight-loss medication. There are now only two weight-loss drugs legally available in the United States for long-term use. One is sibutramine, which is sold under the trade name Meridia. This medication works by suppressing appetite. It

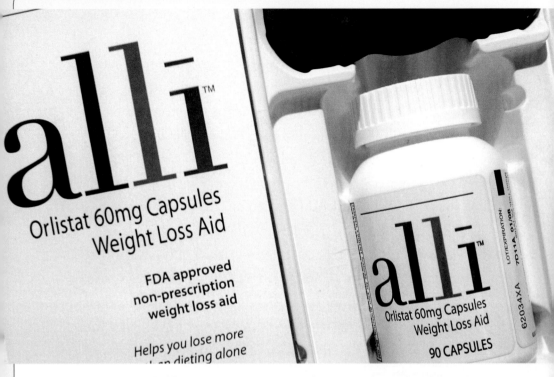

Alli, introduced in 2007, is a lower-dose version of the prescription drug Xenical, which helps block the body's absorption of fat. It is the first over-the-counter weight-loss medication approved by the Food and Drug Administration (FDA).

has some possible side effects, including dry mouth, dizziness, and upset stomach. More seriously, in some people, it causes a sharp increase in blood pressure. High blood pressure can lead to a stroke or a heart attack, so only people with normal blood pressure should take Meridia.

The second weight-loss drug is orlistat, which is marketed under the name Xenical. This medication keeps the intestine from absorbing about one-third of the fat that a person eats. According to the *New York Times*, the average patient taking Xenical loses about 12 pounds (5.4 kg) after six months of taking the drug. Xenical, however, does have a downside. Along with

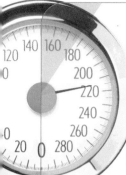

Ten Great Questions to Ask a Doctor

1. What is my BMI, and does it indicate I'm obese?
2. How much weight do I need to lose?
3. What will happen to my body if I don't lose any weight?
4. What type of diet do you recommend?
5. How much exercise should I get daily?
6. What type of exercise do you recommend for me?
7. Do I already have any health problems associated with excess body fat?
8. Should I take a weight-loss drug?
9. Should I consider bariatric surgery?
10. Do you have any advice for me that will increase my chances of weight-loss success?

fat, it inhibits the absorption of certain vitamins and minerals. A person on Xenical, therefore, should take a multivitamin daily. Also, if a patient eats too much fat, he or she might suffer a bout of severe diarrhea.

Given this side effect, it is hardly surprising that many patients have shied away from Xenical. But starting in 2007, the federal government's Food and Drug Administration (FDA) has allowed a lower-dose version of Xenical, called Alli, to be sold in drugstores. This over-the-counter weight-loss medication is the first one that is available without a prescription. Alli has become popular with the public. The *New York Times* reported that more than two million Alli starter kits were sold during its first four months on the market.

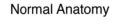

Normal Anatomy

Division of Small Bowel and Stomach

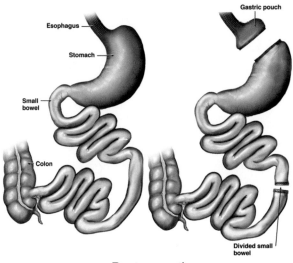

Post-operative Condition

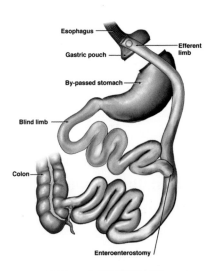

This medical drawing is of the most common type of gastric bypass surgery, which uses the Roux-en-Y procedure. On the top left is the stomach before surgery. The top right picture illustrates how the surgeon creates a small stomach pouch and divides the intestine. On the bottom, the intestine is reconnected to the stomach pouch.

WEIGHT-LOSS SURGERY

For severely obese people with a BMI above 40, a more drastic option is bariatric surgery, also called weight-loss surgery. Bariatric surgery can help a patient lose 100 pounds (45.4 kg) or more. The surgery success stories of celebrities, such as *Today* weatherman Al Roker and singer Carnie Wilson, have heightened interest in this weight-loss method. According to the American Society for Bariatric Surgery, about two hundred thousand weight-loss surgeries were performed in 2007, four times as many as in 2001.

There are several types of bariatric surgery, but the most common is gastric bypass. In this procedure, the surgeon closes off most of the stomach and shortens the small intestine. With the size of the stomach reduced, a person who has had gastric bypass can eat only a very small amount of food at a time, leading to a rapid weight loss.

Another popular bariatric surgery involves the use of a gastric band, also known as the Lap-Band. This inflatable band, made from silicone, is placed around the top part of the stomach to create a small pouch. As in gastric bypass, the reduced stomach fills with food quickly and signals the brain that it is full after only a small meal. Unlike gastric bypass, however, gastric banding surgery does not involve cutting or removing any part of the stomach or intestine. It can also be performed using laparoscopic surgical methods. This means the surgeon does not need to make a big incision into the patient's abdomen. Instead, the surgeon makes a series of tiny cuts, allowing the patient to recover in a shorter period of time.

As with any surgical procedure, the decision to have bariatric surgery is a difficult one. Before the surgery, patients must

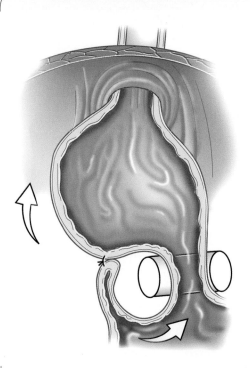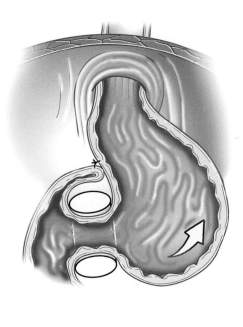

In gastric banding surgery, a band is wrapped around the stomach, creating a small pouch. With the stomach dramatically reduced in size, the post-surgery patient will feel full after only a small meal, allowing the patient to lose weight rapidly.

undergo a program to teach them how to eat and exercise properly post-surgery and to make sure they are psychologically ready for an important lifestyle change. After the surgery, they are monitored by a doctor for the rest of their lives. Bariatric surgery is also very expensive. On average, it costs about thirty thousand dollars for the operation and six months of follow-up care.

Even with the effort and expense involved, more and more Americans are having bariatric surgery each year. For some obese people, it offers a dream come true. The surgery gives them something they may never have had before—the hope that one day they may achieve a normal weight.

Chapter 3

Treating Children and Adolescents

Struggling with weight gain is difficult for anyone. But it is especially hard on one portion of the population—the approximately twenty-five million American children and young adults who are considered overweight or obese. The daily ridicule obese children face from their peers can be devastating to their self-esteem. But far worse is what being so overweight does to their health. Obese children are likely to face severe health problems not only now but also in the future. In December 2007, the *New England Journal of Medicine* reported that the higher a child's BMI is between the ages of seven and thirte, the greater the child's risk will be of developing heart disease as an adult. Findings such as these make the need for understanding the causes of childhood obesity more urgent than ever.

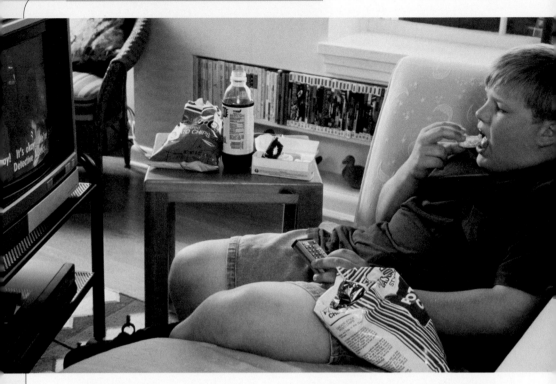

No one knows for certain why the number of overweight children is on the rise in the United States. But two causes cited are constant snacking on junk foods and too much time spent watching TV, rather than engaging in outdoor play.

WHAT MAKES CHILDREN OBESE?

In 2007, the number of overweight children was nearly double what it had been just ten years earlier. No one knows for sure what accounts for this rapid rise. There are plenty of theories, though. Some people blame the changing structure of American family life. In most households, all adults hold down jobs, leaving little time for preparing healthy meals and sitting down together to eat at the dinner table. Older children are frequently left on their own at meal time. Instead of eating a healthy diet, they tend to choose fat-filled fast food, fried snacks, and sugary treats, all loaded with unhealthy calories. Many experts claim that schools are also to blame for children's bad eating habits. School cafeterias often serve soda, pizza, french fries, and other foods that kids may enjoy but that also pack on the pounds.

Others point the finger at children's lack of exercise. At school, fewer and fewer children are enrolled in physical education classes. And at home, parents, afraid to let their children roam their neighborhoods alone, discourage them from playing outside. Stuck inside their homes during most of their playtime, children and adolescents rely on television and video games for entertainment. For hours on end, they sit on a couch looking at a screen, rather than strengthening their bodies and burning calories with outdoor sports and games.

EXAMINING RISK FACTORS

Casting blame is easy. But treating obesity in children and teenagers is very difficult. Sticking with a dietary regime and an exercise plan is a challenge for even the most committed adult. It is not surprising that young people would find it hard to do.

Treating childhood obesity is further complicated by the fact that the field is fairly new. Physicians and teachers, not to mention parents, often do not know how to deal with children's extra weight. To help provide some guidelines, a panel of researchers reviewed current studies into the field and summarized the results in the December 2007 issue of *Pediatrics* magazine.

These researchers found that there are a few behaviors that definitely lead to obesity in children. One is drinking too many

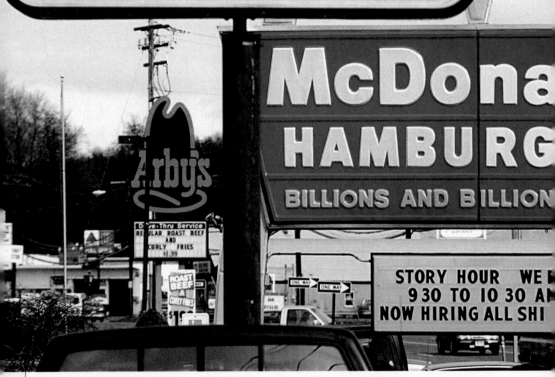

For convenience's sake, many busy families regularly visit fast-food restaurants. Eating meal after meal of high-calorie fast food places both adults and children at risk for obesity. With much of their social life revolving around these inexpensive restaurants, teenagers are especially in danger of overeating fast foods.

sodas and other sugary beverages, such as juice. As reported in *Scientific American*, some obese children consume as many as one thousand calories worth of drinks every day. Not only are these beverages laden with calories, but they also have very little nutritional value.

Young people who skip breakfast are at risk for obesity. Without breakfast, teens especially eat more throughout the day. They are also prone to snacking. Research shows the favorite snacks among teenagers include potato chips, ice cream, candy, cookies, and breakfast cereal. Although these snacks have about the same calorie content as they did in the past, today's teens seem to eat more of them.

Eating a large number of restaurant meals, especially fast food, is also a common habit of obese adolescents. Citing research into this phenomenon, two obese teenagers took McDonald's to court in 2002. They tried unsuccessfully to sue the restaurant giant for their excess weight and their resulting health problems. Fearing similar lawsuits, Burger King and other sellers of fast food have added healthier food to their menus. Even with these options, teenagers still tend to order fatty french fries and hamburgers.

One of the most reliable ways of predicting whether children will become obese is the number of hours of television they watch each day. Television watching not only requires little energy, but it also tends to displace more active play. In other words, the more a young person watches television, the less time he or she has for sports and just playing outside. In addition, many children associate watching television with eating. Television commercials selling sugary and salty snacks, many designed specifically for children, only reinforce this idea.

Weight-Loss Surgery for Teens

Obese teens are increasingly looking to bariatric surgery as a solution to their weight problems. Many surgeons, though, are hesitant to perform weight-loss surgeries on young people. Their bodies are often still growing, and sometimes teenagers are not mature enough to truly commit to the lifelong eating and exercise plans needed for success. In addition, researchers know little about the long-term health effects of weight-loss surgery on adolescents.

NEW STRATEGIES

These findings suggest a few simple things parents can do to help their obese children lose weight. They can stop buying soda or limit their kids' television time. (The American Academy of Pediatrics suggests children watch no more than two hours each day.) With the help of a physician, parents can also set goals for their children's weight loss. Offering small gifts and other rewards can be effective in motivating children to work toward these goals.

The CDC suggests parents show their children how to eat right by eating right themselves. It also encourages parents to organize their family time around outdoor play and other physical activities. According to the U.S. Department of Agriculture (USDA), children need at least sixty minutes of moderate exercise every day.

be our guest and enjoy a

FREE
KIDS MEAL

579 JONESBORO RD
MCDONOUGH, GA 30252
678-583-1998

4980 BILL GARDNER PKWY
LOCUST GROVE, GA 30248
678-583-8186

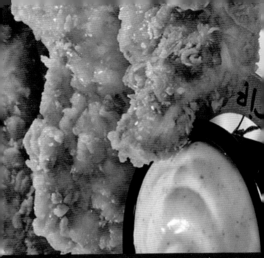

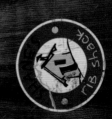

FREE
Kids Meal

rib shack

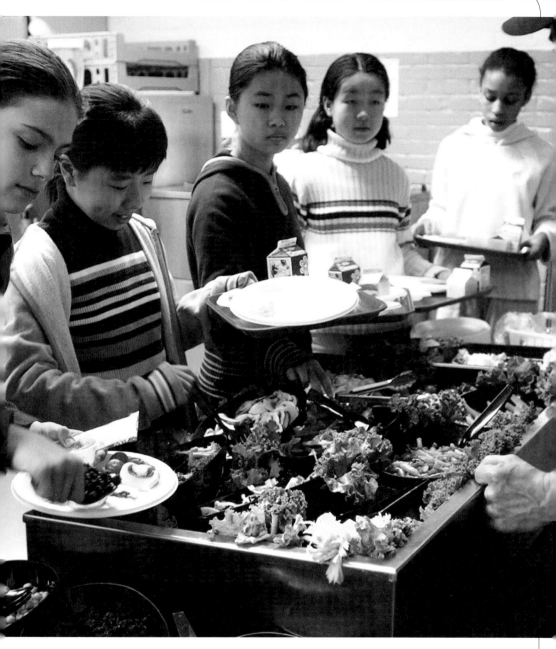

Students at a Connecticut middle school line up for the salad bar in their lunchroom. School cafeterias throughout the United States are banishing fatty foods, such as burgers and pizza, while also encouraging young people to eat more fruits and vegetables.

Many parents complain that obesity report cards give them nothing but numbers. They may be told their children are obese, but they are not given any information or help in deciding what to do about it. At worst, issuing obesity report cards seems a way for schools to act as though they are dealing with childhood obesity without actually doing anything at all. As David Ludwig, director of the Optimal Weight for Life program at Children's Hospital in Boston told the *New York Times* in 2007, "It would be the height of irony if we successfully identified overweight kids through BMI screening and notification while continuing to feed them atrocious quality meals and snacks, with limited if any opportunities for phys ed in school."

Chapter 4

The Dark Side of Obesity Treatment

Anyone who has lost weight knows it is difficult to keep from regaining it. Researchers have also found that the opposite is true. If thin people purposely try to gain weight, it is hard for them to keep on the extra pounds, even if they continue to overeat. Based on such research, weight-loss experts have theorized that people tend to have a natural weight range, which may be as small as 10 to 20 pounds (4.5 to 9 kg). No matter how much or how little a person eats, the body will resist going above or below that range.

It would seem this idea should discourage anyone from trying to drastically lower their weight. But Americans are an optimistic people, confident they can do whatever they set their minds on. According to Marketdata Enterprise, which studies the weight-loss market, about seventy-two million Americans are on a diet at any given time.

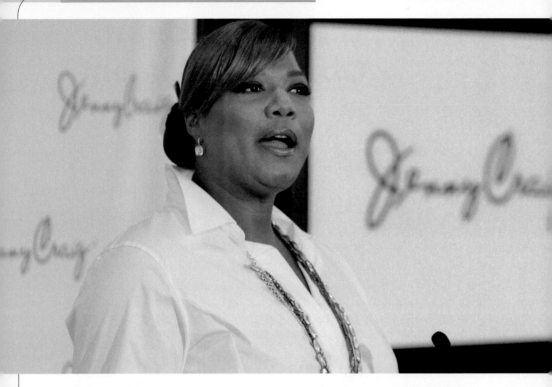

Actress and singer Queen Latifah announces her plans to go on the Jenny Craig weight-loss program during a 2008 press conference. Celebrity endorsements are often used by the weight-loss industry to encourage dieters to try their products.

Risky Weight Loss

With so many people dieting, there is an enormous demand for weight-loss products—from meal replacement bars to diet soda to over-the-counter weight-loss pills. In fact, Marketdata estimates Americans spend some fifty-five billion dollars on the weight-loss industry each year. With that much money on the line, weight-loss companies go to great lengths to convince discouraged dieters that their product is the one that will finally let them lose those extra pounds. Their advertisements make big promises, often featuring dramatic before and after pictures and celebrity endorsements. Many of the products are worthless, though. Customers who think they are buying a weight-loss miracle get nothing for their money except false hope.

Some diet products are worse than useless. They are actually dangerous. For example, herbal weight-loss pills, also known as nutritionals, do not have to be approved by the Food and Drug Administration (FDA). (This government agency tests drugs to make sure they are safe.) Taken alone or with other drugs, a few nutritionals have proven to be a health hazard. One recent example is ephedra. Ephedra was sold as a weight-loss supplement until 2004, when it was banned by the FDA. A year earlier, Steve Bechler, a baseball player for the Baltimore Orioles, died of heatstroke. He had been taking ephedra, which was found to be partially responsible for his death.

Even drugs approved by the FDA have been known to cause health problems. In the 1990s, a combination of two drugs (fenfluramine and phentermine) became known as fen-phen. Fen-phen, prescribed as an obesity medication, was enormously popular. But in July 1997, researchers at the Mayo Clinic reported that twenty-four women taking fen-phen had developed a rare heart valve abnormality. After other similar cases came to light, the FDA took fen-phen off the market.

More recently, some experts have become concerned about the safety of bariatric surgery. The death rate from weight-loss surgery had been estimated at under 1 percent. But a 2005 study published by the *Journal of the American Medical Association* showed that among thirty-five- to forty-five-year-olds, the rate of death within a year after the surgery was more than 5 percent for men and nearly 3 percent for women. In addition, four out of every ten patients suffer complications within six months. These

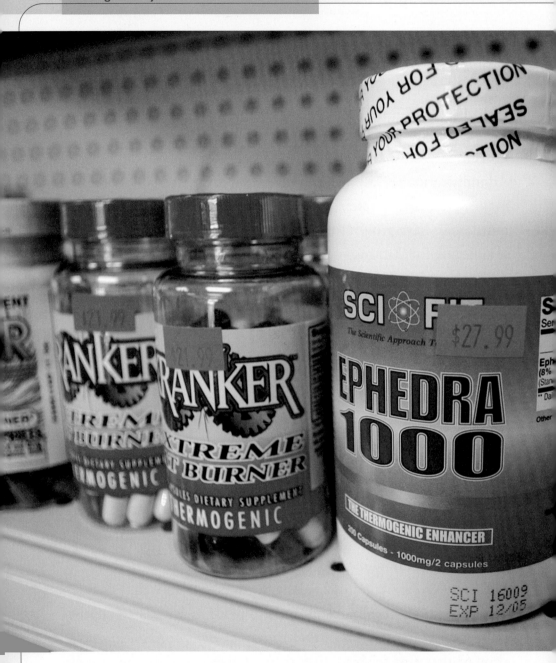

Ephedra was a traditional herbal medicine used in China for thousands of years. Until 2004, it was sold in the United States as a dietary supplement used for losing weight. That same year, it was banned by the FDA in response to a number of ephedra-related deaths, most notably that of Baltimore Orioles pitcher Steve Bechler in 2003.

complications include vomiting, infection, and leaking surgical connections between the stomach and intestines. Sometimes, the problems are serious enough to require rehospitalization or even additional surgery.

With the popularity of weight-loss surgery, many surgeons have moved into this lucrative field. Bariatric surgery is challenging, though. Surgeons new to gastric bypass essentially have to master the operation on the job, which can prove dangerous to their patients. In 2007, the *New York Times* reported on a study that discovered doctors' first nineteen bariatric surgery patients were five times more likely to die than their patients on whom they later performed the surgery.

EMBRACING FAT

Death on the operating table is certainly scary to obesity patients, but even relatively safe weight-loss methods can have their hazards. One is the phenomenon called yo-yo dieting. Yo-yo dieters fall into a pattern of dieting to lose weight, only to gain back all of it and perhaps a few additional pounds as well, spurring them on to diet again. This constant cycle of losing and gaining can cause wear and tear on the body. It can also do a good deal of psychological damage. With their weight, the emotions of yo-yo dieters go up and down. They feel elated when they are losing weight, only to feel devastated when the weight comes back. Dieters are often left with an unresolved weight problem and a gnawing sense of failure.

In addition, yo-yo dieting is frequently a financial strain. In each cycle, dieters grow more determined to do it right this time.

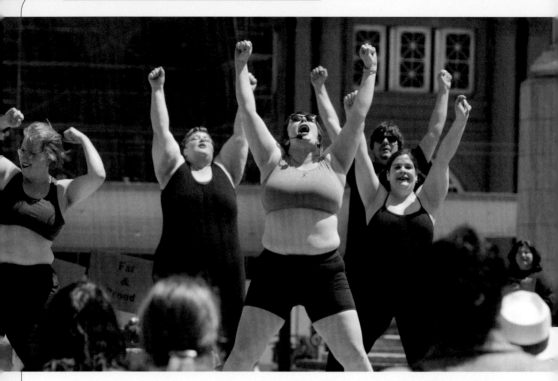

Jennifer Portnick (in the blue top) and other activists perform an aerobics routine in 2002 on No Diet Day—an international event held every May 6 to promote fat acceptance. Portnick filed a discrimination complaint against a dance fitness program, after it refused to hire her as an instructor because of her size.

They can fall prey to marketing pitches for obesity products that appeal to their desperation for weight-loss success.

To some obese people, the physical and mental toll of dieting hardly seems worth it. Beginning in the 1990s, a group of people joined together to organize the grassroots Fat Acceptance Movement. Its members call themselves "fat," using the word with pride. They challenge the negative stereotypes associated with being overweight and work to fight the discrimination many obese people face in society. Many obese people also question the medical community's insistence that being fat is the same thing as being unhealthy. Some overweight activists insist that their extra pounds do not necessarily mean that their bodies are not physically fit.

MEDICINE AND THE WEIGHT-LOSS INDUSTRY

The "fat can be fit" argument was bolstered by a 2005 study authored by Katherine M. Flegel at the Centers for Disease Control and Prevention. Flegel analyzed data from a national survey on obesity and came to a surprising conclusion. She found that mildly overweight adults had a lower risk of dying than adults at a normal weight.

The novelty of the idea attracted the national press, which quickly picked up the story. Just as fast, obesity experts moved to attack Flegel's findings. Especially vocal were researchers at the Harvard School of Public Health, who over the past decades have been largely responsible for publicizing the health risks of obesity. The Harvard researchers launched a well-organized attack on Flegel's findings. They even held a special conference just to refute Flegel's study.

The swift and furious reaction to Flegel's work revealed another challenge America faces in understanding obesity. Just like the weight-loss product industry, many research centers, drug companies, hospitals, and government-run health agencies have a great deal invested in presenting obesity as an enormous public health crisis. This idea attracts a large amount of funding, which is often spent on informing the public about the obesity epidemic and instructing them how to diet and exercise to prevent weight gain. Quoted in Gina Kolata's *Rethinking Thin*, obesity expert Jeffrey Friedman explains how this can inhibit a prejudice-free examination of obesity, its causes, and its treatment: "A lot of the reasons that perceptions about obesity are slow to change is that there is a huge financial and personal interest on the part of many promoting the message that 'this is your fault.' That includes the diet industry and a subgroup of the, quote, scientific community whose careers are invested in the idea that you can implement a set of behavioral measures that can treat obesity."

Chapter 5

The Future of Obesity Treatment

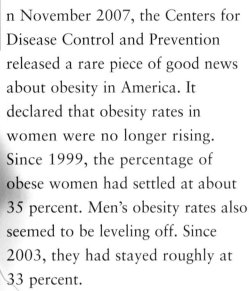

In November 2007, the Centers for Disease Control and Prevention released a rare piece of good news about obesity in America. It declared that obesity rates in women were no longer rising. Since 1999, the percentage of obese women had settled at about 35 percent. Men's obesity rates also seemed to be leveling off. Since 2003, they had stayed roughly at 33 percent.

Another bright spot in obesity treatment is the number of promising new therapies on the horizon. With so many people desperate for help with their weight problems, researchers are understandably driven to find new ways to fight obesity. Rather than searching for a miracle diet, though, many are asking a very basic question: could there be something wrong in the bodies of some people that make them obese?

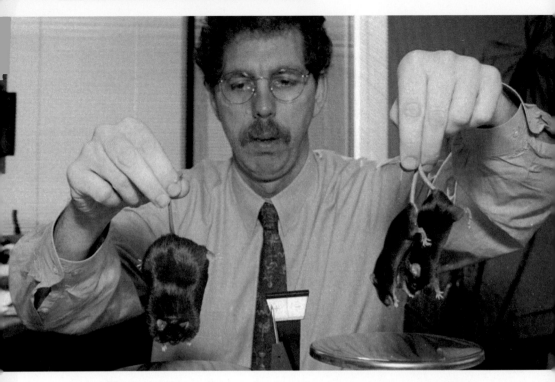

Scientist Jeffrey Friedman weighs one obese mouse and two slim ones as part of his ongoing research into the causes of obesity. In 1994, he discovered that the bodies of very fat mice lacked a hormone called leptin, which caused them to be constantly hungry.

LEPTIN AND OBESITY

In 1994, researcher Jeffrey Friedman found a partial answer to this question. Experimenting on very fat mice, he found that their bodies lacked a protein hormone called leptin. Because of their lack of leptin, the mice were always hungry. Trying to satisfy their never-ending desire for food, they ate constantly.

Friedman then injected the mice with leptin and watched what happened. The hormone not only reduced their appetite but also helped them burn energy. With regular leptin injections, the obese mice slimmed down fast.

Eating and Addiction

Scientists studying compulsive overeaters have made an interesting discovery. In some ways, their brains are similar to those of drug addicts. Both groups seem to have an abnormal response to dopamine—a hormone associated with feelings of pleasure. Both eating and taking illegal drugs, such as cocaine, release dopamine. Perhaps people who do these activities compulsively are unknowingly driven by a need to increase their low dopamine levels.

This theory could lead to new treatments for overeaters. Scientists are trying to create drugs designed to increase dopamine levels and thus remove the urge to binge. Weight-loss counselors are also recognizing that, like addicts, overeaters can often benefit from group therapy.

The discovery excited scientists studying obesity. Could a lack of leptin account for obesity in humans? Could leptin injections also bring obese people to a normal weight? Unfortunately, the answer was no. Later experiments showed only a very few obese people could benefit from leptin injections. Friedman's research did suggest that the high rate of obesity might be caused by something other than too much eating and not enough exercise. Maybe there was something amiss in the bodies of obese people that someday science could fix.

Researchers are also asking another question: is there something about the bodies of normal-weight people that helps keep them that way? One area of research studies the trillions of tiny organisms called microbes that are found in everyone's stomach.

These microbes help break down food. There are different types of microbes, and they do not all act in the same manner. Researchers at Washington University in St. Louis have discovered that, in the stomachs of thin people, there are often a large number of one type of microbes called *Bacterioidetes*. These bacteria might help break down food in a way that keeps it from getting turned into fat.

A Revolution in Drug Treatment

Another intriguing area of study revolves around ghrelin. This hormone is found in the stomach and spurs appetite. Gastric bypass helps people lose weight, not only by reducing the size of the stomach but probably also by lowering levels of ghrelin. Scientists are now using what they know about ghrelin to try to create an anti-obesity vaccine.

Scientists are also working to create new and better obesity drugs. In fact, there are at least two hundred possible drug therapies now being studied. Creating new obesity drugs is challenging, though. The body's regulation of energy involves the brain and many other organs. Any drug that alters it is likely to affect other bodily processes, producing unwanted side effects.

For instance, American researchers had high hopes for a medicine called rimonabant. Sold under the name Acomplia in Europe, rimonabant suppresses appetite, helping obese patients lose as much as 5 percent of their body weight. Unfortunately, it also doubles a person's risk of severe anxiety and depression. Citing these side effects, a federal advisory panel voted against its sale in the United States in 2007. The Food and Drug Administration is unlikely to approve rimonabant anytime soon.

Despite this setback, some experts predict that eventually obesity will be treated with a variety of drugs. Doctors may prescribe several drugs for the same patient, much as they do now to treat high blood pressure and diabetes.

NEW WAYS OF LOOKING AT OBESITY

Our current obesity treatments largely focus on changing people's behavior. But increasingly, scientists are suggesting that obesity does not have its roots in how much people eat and exercise. Many believe that some people's bodies might be programmed at birth to become obese.

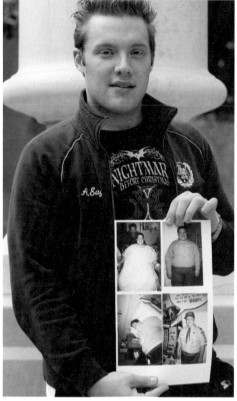

At the age of seventeen, Eric Decker lost weight through surgery. One day, science might give obese teens a less drastic option.

In 2006, researchers at Boston University made an interesting discovery. They discovered a common variation in the human genetic code. According to the journal *Science*, this variant is found in about 10 percent of people of European and African American descent. Research shows that this inherited trait makes a person much more likely to gain weight. If both parents have it, the probability that that person will be obese rises by 22 percent. This is just one way the field of genetics will likely change the

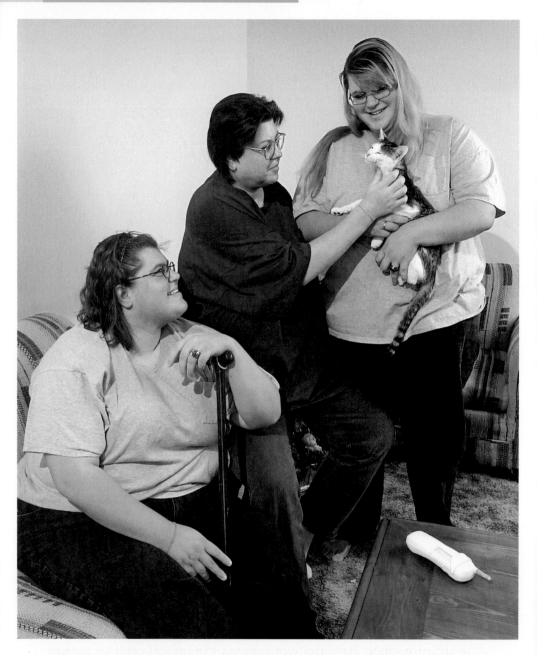

Twins Tanya and Trisha Hence, shown here with their mother, struggled with obesity before undergoing gastric bypass surgery in 2002. One year after their surgery, the twins lost a combined 272 pounds (123 kg). Many studies, including some involving twins, have shown that people can inherit a tendency to gain weight and become obese.

Zapping Fat

A company called Medtronic is testing a new way to help people lose weight. It manufactures a gastric stimulator. About the size of a pocket watch, this device can be surgically implanted in the stomach of an obese patient. The stimulator then sends out a series of electrical pulses. The pulses trick the brain into thinking the stomach is full, even when it is not. They may also be able slow the rate of digestion, resulting in further weight loss. The gastric stimulator is not yet approved for sale in the United States, but it has been available in Europe since 2001.

way we look at extra weight. Scientists may find out more links between genes and obesity in the near future.

Some researchers theorize that a tendency toward obesity can set in during early childhood, or even in the womb. For instance, one study looked at children of women who had untreated diabetes during their pregnancy. Between the ages of five and seven, those children were twice as likely to be obese than children of healthy mothers.

Other scientists speculate that increases in obesity rates are part of a bigger picture. In many ways, human beings are changing. For example, on average, people are taller and smarter (as measured by IQ) than they were even in the recent past. Perhaps their becoming heavier is merely part of this trend. Extra weight might just be the result of better nutrition in mothers and infants or of vaccines that prevent certain illnesses early in life. These ideas suggest that a new diet or a perfect exercise plan might not be the right place to look for a "cure" for obesity. More likely, as scientists learn more about obesity and the body, they will find new and unexpected solutions to this challenging problem.

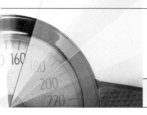

Glossary

bariatric surgery Surgery performed to aid a patient in losing weight. The word "bariatric" means "relating to the treatment of obesity."

behavioral therapy A treatment program that involves substituting desirable behavioral responses for undersirable responses.

body fat Body tissue that stores energy.

body mass index (BMI) A measure of body fat calculated from a person's height and weight.

calorie A unit of measurement equal to the amount of energy needed to increase the temperature of 1 kilogram of water by 1 degree Celsius.

diabetes A disease in which a person either doesn't make insulin (a hormone needed for the cells to use sugar from foods) or doesn't use it properly.

discrimination Prejudicial and unequal treatment of a person or group of people.

fad diet An eating plan promising extraordinary weight loss that enjoys a brief period of popularity and usually relies on peculiar food choices.

gastric band surgery A bariatric surgical technique in which a surgeon places an inflatable silicone band around the top part of the stomach to reduce its size.

gastric bypass A bariatric surgical technique in which a surgeon closes off most of the stomach and shortens the small intestine.

laparoscopic surgery A surgical technique in which operations are performed by making a series of tiny cuts instead of large incisions.

leptin A hormone that regulates appetite.

obese Having a BMI of 30 or more.

orlistat An obesity drug, marketed under the names Xenical and Alli, that prevents the body from absorbing some dietary fat.

overweight Having a BMI between 25 and 29.9.

sibutramine An obesity drug, marketed under the name Meridia, that suppresses appetite.

very low-calorie diet (VLCD) A weight-loss eating plan that restricts the daily calorie intake to 800 or less.

yo-yo dieting Eating habit characterized by periods of weight loss alternating with periods of weight gain.

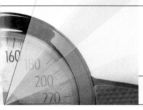

For More Information

Canadian Obesity Network
Royal Alexandra Hospital
Room 102, Materials Management Centre
10240 Kingsway Avenue
Edmonton, AB T5H 3V9
Canada
(289) 238-9148
Web site: http://www.obesitynetwork.ca
Affiliated with McMaster University, the Canadian Obesity Network sponsors
workshops and conferences that bring together some two thousand obesity
researchers and health professionals working in Canada.

Centers for Disease Control and Prevention
1600 Clifton Road
Atlanta, GA 30333
(888) 232-6348
Web site: http://www.cdc.gov/nccdphp/dnpa/obesity/index.htm
A federal agency charged with protecting public health, the Centers for Disease
Control and Prevention studies the causes and treatments of obesity, which
it summarizes on the "Overweight and Obesity" section on its Web site.

**Harvard Prevention Research Center on Nutrition
and Physical Activity**
Harvard School of Public Health
677 Huntington Avenue, 7th Floor
Boston, MA 02115

(617) 432-3840

Web site: http://www.hsph.harvard.edu/prc

The Harvard Prevention Research Center develops programs to reduce childhood obesity by promoting improved nutrition and increased physical activity.

MyPyramid

USDA Center for Nutrition Policy and Promotion

3101 Park Center Drive

Room 1034

Alexandria, VA 22302

(888) 779-7264

Web site: http://www.pyramid.gov

Sponsored by the U.S. Department of Agriculture, MyPyramid offers dieters free personalized eating and exercise plans through its Web site.

National Association to Advance Fat Acceptance

P.O. Box 22510

Oakland, CA 94609

(916) 558-6880

Web site: http://www.naafa.org

Founded in 1969, NAAFA is a nonprofit organization dedicated to improving the lives of "fat people" through promoting self-respect and offering public education about size discrimination.

National Weight Control Registry

Brown Medical School/The Miriam Hospital

Weight Control & Diabetes Research Center

196 Richmond Street

Providence, RI 02903

(800) 606-6927

Web site: http://www.nwcr.ws

By tracking the progress of more than five thousand people who have lost
weight and kept it off, the National Weight Control Registry is devoted
to developing practical strategies for weight loss and weight control.

We Can!

National Heart, Lung, and Blood Institute

NHLBI Health Information Center

P.O. Box 30105

Bethesda, MD 20824

(301) 592-8573

Web site: http://www.nhlbi.nih.gov/health/public/heart/
obesity/wecan

Standing for "ways to enhance children's activity and nutrition," We Can!
offers people tips about how to help children maintain a healthy weight.

Web Sites

Due to the changing nature of Internet links, Rosen Publishing
has developed an online list of Web sites related to the subject of
this book. This site is updated regularly. Please use this link to
access the list:

http://www.rosenlinks.com/uno/trob

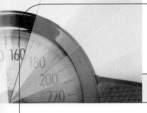

For Further Reading

Akers, Charlene. *Obesity*. San Diego, CA: Lucent Books, 2000.

Ford, Jean, and Autumn Libal. *The Truth About Diets: The Pros and Cons*. Philadelphia, PA: Mason Crest Publishers, 2005.

Gay, Kathlyn. *Am I Fat? The Obesity Issue for Teens*. Berkeley Heights, NJ: Enslow Publishers, 2006.

Harmon, Daniel E. *Obesity* (Coping in a Changing World). New York, NY: Rosen Publishing, 2007.

Hunter, William. *Medications and Surgeries for Weight Loss: When Dieting Isn't Enough*. Philadelphia, PA: Mason Crest Publishers, 2005.

Ingram, Scott. *Want Fries with That? Obesity and the Supersizing of America*. New York, NY: Franklin Watts, 2005.

Kolata, Gina. *Rethinking Thin: The New Science of Weight Loss— and the Myths and Realities of Dieting*. New York, NY: Farrar, Straus and Giroux, 2007.

Libal, Autumn. *The Importance of Physical Activity and Exercise: The Fitness Factor*. Philadelphia, PA: Mason Crest Publishers, 2005.

National Institutes of Health. *The Practical Guide: Identification, Evaluation, and Treatment of Overweight and Obesity in Adults*. Retrieved December 14, 2007 (http://www.nhlbi.nih. gov/guidelines/obesity/prctgd_b.pdf).

Owens, Peter. *Teens Health & Obesity*. Philadelphia, PA: Mason Crest Publishers, 2005.

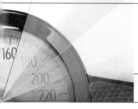

Bibliography

Fletcher, Anne M. *Thin for Life: 10 Keys to Success from People Who Have Lost Weight and Kept It Off*. Boston, MA: Houghton Mifflin, 2003.

Kolata, Gina. *Rethinking Thin: The New Science of Weight Loss—and the Myths and Realities of Dieting*. New York, NY: Farrar, Straus and Giroux, 2007.

National Institutes of Health. *The Practical Guide: Identification, Evaluation, and Treatment of Overweight and Obesity in Adults*. Retrieved December 14, 2007 (http://www.nhlbi.nih.gov/guidelines/obesity/prctgd_b.pdf).

Nestle, Marion. "Eating Made Simple." *Scientific American*, Vol. 297, No. 3, September 2007, pp. 60–69.

Raeburn, Paul. "Can Fit Be Fat." *Scientific American*, Vol. 297, No. 3, September 2007, pp. 70–71.

Spear, Bonnie A., et al. "Recommendations for Treatment of Child and Adolescent Overweight and Obesity." *Pediatrics*, Vol. 120, December 2007, pp. 254–288.

Wadden, Thomas A., and Albert J. Stunkard, eds. *Handbook of Obesity Treatment*. New York, NY: Guilford Press, 2002.

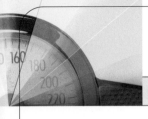

Index

About the Author

A graduate of Swarthmore College, Liz Sonneborn is a full-time writer living in Brooklyn, New York. She has written more than sixty non-fiction books for teens and adults on a wide variety of subjects. Her books dealing with science include *Forces in Nature: Understanding Gravitational, Electrical, and Magnetic Force*; *Guglielmo Marconi: Inventor of Wireless Technology*; and *The Electric Light: Thomas Edison's Illuminating Invention*. After years of reading articles and journals about nutrition and fitness, Sonneborn found researching obesity and its treatment fascinating. As she explains, "It is clear the old diet-and-exercise advice is not helping most obese people get control of their weight. Willpower is only part, and possibly a small part, of the answer to this country's obesity problem. I suspect and hope that, in the years to come, scientific research will provide better solutions."

Photo Credits

Editor: Kathy Kuhtz Campbell; Photo Researcher: Cindy Reiman